Delicious Recipes to Beat Gout

Your Ultimate Gout Diet Cookbook for a Pain-Free Life!

T. John

COPYRIGHT PAGE

TABLE OF CONTENTS

Chapter 8: Beverages for Gout Management

Chapter 9: Meal Planning and Tips for Gout-Friendly Eating

INTRODUCTION

Once upon a time, in a world where the hustle and bustle of modern life often leaves little time for self-care, a group of health-conscious individuals found themselves facing a common foe - gout. Gout, a type of arthritis characterized by sudden and severe joint pain, often caused by the accumulation of uric acid crystals, had become an unwelcome guest in their lives. As they searched for ways to manage this condition and improve their overall well-being, they stumbled upon a treasure trove of delicious recipes that could help them beat gout and lead a more vibrant, pain-free life.

And so, the idea for the book "Delicious Recipes to Beat Gout" was born. This comprehensive guide, compiled by a team of culinary enthusiasts and health experts, aims to provide a roadmap for those who are looking to harness the power of food in their fight against gout. With a focus on mouthwatering recipes that are not only nutritious but also full of flavor, this book promises to be a game-changer for anyone seeking to take control of their gout management journey.

But before we dive into the tantalizing recipes that await, let's take a moment to understand the basics of gout, its causes, symptoms, and risk factors. Knowledge is power, and arming ourselves with the right information can pave the way for a more informed and effective approach towards managing this condition.

Chapter 1: Understanding Gout

Gout is a form of arthritis that has been affecting humans for centuries. It is a painful condition that is caused by the accumulation of uric acid crystals in joints, leading to inflammation, swelling, and severe pain. Gout most commonly affects the big toe, but it can also affect other joints such as the ankles, knees, elbows, wrists, and fingers. The excruciating pain associated with gout can be debilitating and severely impact a person's quality of life.

In recent years, there has been growing awareness about the role of diet in managing gout. Research has shown that certain foods and dietary habits can trigger gout attacks, while others can help prevent them. In this comprehensive guide, we will delve into the causes, symptoms, and risk factors of gout, explore the importance of diet in managing gout, and how delicious recipes can play a crucial role in beating gout.

Causes of Gout

Gout is caused by the accumulation of uric acid in the blood, a waste product that is normally filtered out by the kidneys and excreted in urine. When the body produces too much uric acid or fails to excrete it efficiently, the uric acid can form crystals that deposit in the joints, leading to inflammation and pain.

There are several factors that can contribute to the development of gout, including:

1. Diet: Consuming foods that are high in purines, which are naturally occurring compounds found in certain foods, can increase the production of uric acid in the body. Foods that are particularly high in purines include organ meats (such as liver, kidneys, and sweetbreads), red meat, seafood (such as anchovies, sardines, mackerel, and scallops), and some types of vegetables (such as asparagus, mushrooms, and spinach).

2. Genetics: Gout can also run in families, indicating a genetic predisposition to the condition. If you have a

family history of gout, you may be at a higher risk of developing it yourself.

3. Obesity: Being overweight or obese can increase the risk of developing gout. Excess body weight can lead to higher levels of uric acid in the blood and put additional pressure on the joints, increasing the risk of gout attacks.

4. Medical conditions: Certain medical conditions, such as high blood pressure, diabetes, kidney disease, and metabolic syndrome, can increase the risk of developing gout.

5. Medications: Some medications, such as diuretics (used to treat high blood pressure) and low-dose aspirin, can increase the levels of uric acid in the blood and trigger gout attacks.

Symptoms of Gout

Gout typically presents with sudden and severe pain in the affected joint, along with other symptoms such as:

- Swelling, redness, and warmth in the affected joint
- Tenderness and sensitivity to touch

- Limited range of motion in the joint
- Skin over the joint may appear shiny and stretched

Gout attacks can occur suddenly and usually peak within 24 hours. The pain can be so intense that even the slightest touch or movement can cause excruciating discomfort. Gout attacks often occur at night and can last for several days to weeks.

It's important to note that not everyone with high levels of uric acid in their blood will develop gout, and not all gout attacks are the same. Some people may experience mild gout attacks with less severe symptoms, while others may have frequent and severe gout attacks that significantly impact their daily lives.

Risk Factors for Gout

There are several risk factors that can increase the likelihood of developing gout, including:

1. Gender and age: Gout is more common in men than women, and the risk of developing gout increases

with age. Men typically develop gout after the age of 30, while women are at a higher risk after menopause.

2. Family history: If you have a family history of gout, you may be more likely to develop the condition yourself, indicating a genetic predisposition.

3. Diet: Consuming a diet that is high in purine-rich foods, as mentioned earlier, can increase the risk of developing gout. Additionally, consuming high amounts of fructose, found in sugary beverages and foods, has also been linked to an increased risk of gout.

4. Alcohol consumption: Regular and excessive alcohol consumption, particularly of beer, has been associated with a higher risk of developing gout. Alcohol can increase the production of uric acid in the body and decrease its excretion, leading to higher levels of uric acid in the blood.

5. Medical conditions: Certain medical conditions, such as kidney disease, high blood pressure, diabetes, and metabolic syndrome, can increase the risk of developing gout.

6. Medications: Some medications, such as diuretics (used to treat high blood pressure), low-dose aspirin, and certain immunosuppressive drugs, can increase the levels of uric acid in the blood and trigger gout attacks.

Importance of Diet in Managing Gout

Diet plays a crucial role in managing gout. Making appropriate dietary changes can help reduce the production of uric acid in the body, promote its excretion, and prevent the formation of uric acid crystals in the joints, thereby reducing the frequency and severity of gout attacks.

In this section, we will delve into the dietary recommendations for managing gout, including:

1. Purine-rich foods to avoid: Certain foods that are high in purines should be limited or avoided in a gout-friendly diet. These include organ meats, red meat, seafood, and some types of vegetables, as mentioned earlier.

2. High-fructose foods to limit: Foods that are high in fructose, such as sugary beverages and foods, should also be limited as they have been associated with increased uric acid production in the body.

3. Alcohol moderation: Limiting or avoiding alcohol consumption, particularly of beer, can help manage gout as alcohol can increase uric acid production and reduce its excretion.

4. Hydration: Staying well-hydrated by drinking plenty of water can help promote the excretion of uric acid through urine, reducing the risk of gout attacks.

5. Low-fat dairy products: Low-fat dairy products, such as milk, yogurt, and cheese, have been shown to have a protective effect against gout as they can help lower uric acid levels in the blood.

6. High-fiber foods: Consuming foods that are high in fiber, such as whole grains, fruits, and vegetables, can help lower uric acid levels in the blood and promote overall health.

7. Weight management: Maintaining a healthy weight through regular exercise and a balanced diet can help

reduce the risk of developing gout or managing existing gout.

Chapter 2: Gout-Friendly Breakfast Recipes

Breakfast is the most important meal of the day, and it sets the tone for your overall health and well-being. By starting your day with gout-friendly breakfast recipes, you can kickstart your day on the right note, and also support your gout management goals. In this chapter, we will explore some delicious and nutritious breakfast recipes that are low in purines and can help you beat gout while still enjoying a flavorful morning meal.

Hearty Quinoa Breakfast Bowl

Ingredients:

- 1 cup cooked quinoa
- 1/2 cup diced bell peppers (red, yellow, and/or green)
- 1/2 cup diced zucchini
- 1/4 cup diced red onion
- 1 clove garlic, minced
- 1 tablespoon olive oil
- 1/2 teaspoon dried oregano

- Salt and pepper to taste
- 2 large eggs
- Fresh parsley for garnish (optional)

Directions:

1. Heat olive oil in a pan over medium heat. Add minced garlic and sauté for 1 minute.
2. Add diced bell peppers, zucchini, and red onion to the pan. Sauté for 3-4 minutes until the vegetables are slightly softened.
3. Add cooked quinoa, dried oregano, salt, and pepper to the pan. Stir-fry for another 2-3 minutes until the flavors meld together.
4. Create two wells in the quinoa mixture and crack an egg into each well. Cover the pan and let the eggs cook for 3-4 minutes until the whites are set but the yolks are still slightly runny.
5. Garnish with fresh parsley (if desired) and serve hot as a delicious and protein-packed breakfast bowl.

Veggie and Egg Breakfast Skillet

Ingredients:

- 1 tablespoon olive oil
- 1/2 cup diced bell peppers (red, yellow, and/or green)
- 1/2 cup diced zucchini
- 1/4 cup diced red onion
- 1 clove garlic, minced
- 2 large eggs
- Salt and pepper to taste
- Fresh basil for garnish (optional)

Directions:

1. Heat olive oil in a skillet over medium heat. Add minced garlic and sauté for 1 minute.
2. Add diced bell peppers, zucchini, and red onion to the skillet. Sauté for 3-4 minutes until the vegetables are slightly softened.
3. Create two wells in the vegetable mixture and crack an egg into each well. Sprinkle with salt and pepper.

4. Cover the skillet and let the eggs cook for 3-4 minutes until the whites are set but the yolks are still slightly runny.

5. Garnish with fresh basil (if desired) and serve hot as a nutritious and flavorful breakfast skillet.

Spinach and Mushroom Omelette

Ingredients:

- 3 large eggs
- 1 cup fresh spinach leaves, chopped
- 1/2 cup sliced mushrooms
- 1/4 cup diced red onion
- 1 clove garlic, minced
- 1 tablespoon olive oil
- Salt and pepper to taste
- 1/4 cup shredded low-fat cheese (such as mozzarella or Swiss)
- Fresh parsley for garnish (optional)

Directions:

1. In a bowl, beat the eggs with salt and pepper.

2. Heat olive oil in a non-stick skillet over medium heat. Add minced garlic and sauté for 1 minute.

3. Add diced red onion and sliced mushrooms to the skillet. Sauté for 3-4 minutes until the vegetables are softened.

4. Add chopped spinach to the skillet and sauté for another 2-3 minutes until wilted.

5. Pour the beaten eggs over the vegetables in the skillet. Cook for 2-3 minutes until the edges are set.

6. Sprinkle shredded cheese over one half of the omelette. Fold the other half over the cheese and cook for another 1-2 minutes until the cheese is melted and the omelette is cooked through.

7. Slide the omelette onto a plate, garnish with fresh parsley (if desired), and serve hot as a delicious and protein-packed breakfast option.

Avocado and Tomato Toast

Ingredients:

- 2 slices of whole-grain bread
- 1 ripe avocado, mashed

- 1 small tomato, sliced
- 1 clove garlic, minced
- 1 tablespoon lemon juice
- Salt and pepper to taste
- Fresh basil for garnish (optional)

Directions:

1. Toast the slices of whole-grain bread until crispy.
2. In a bowl, mix mashed avocado with minced garlic, lemon juice, salt, and pepper.
3. Spread the avocado mixture evenly onto the toasted bread slices.
4. Top with sliced tomatoes and garnish with fresh basil (if desired).
5. Serve as a nutrient-rich and satisfying breakfast toast option.

Sweet Potato and Turkey Sausage Hash

Ingredients:

- 1 large sweet potato, peeled and diced
- 1/2 pound lean turkey sausage, crumbled
- 1/2 cup diced bell peppers (red, yellow, and/or green)
- 1/4 cup diced red onion
- 2 cloves garlic, minced
- 2 tablespoons olive oil
- Salt and pepper to taste
- Fresh cilantro for garnish (optional)

Directions:

1. In a large skillet, heat olive oil over medium heat. Add minced garlic and sauté for 1 minute.
2. Add diced sweet potatoes to the skillet and cook for 5-7 minutes, stirring occasionally, until the sweet potatoes are slightly softened.
3. Add crumbled turkey sausage, diced bell peppers, and red onion to the skillet. Cook for another 5-7 minutes, stirring occasionally, until the sausage is cooked through and the vegetables are tender.
4. Season with salt and pepper to taste.

5. Garnish with fresh cilantro (if desired) and serve hot as a flavorful and protein-packed breakfast hash.

Greek Yogurt and Berry Smoothie

Ingredients:

- 1 cup Greek yogurt
- 1/2 cup mixed berries (such as strawberries, blueberries, and raspberries)
- 1 small banana
- 1 tablespoon honey or maple syrup
- 1/2 cup milk (any type)
- 1/2 teaspoon vanilla extract
- Ice cubes (optional)

Directions:

1. Place Greek yogurt, mixed berries, banana, honey or maple syrup, milk, and vanilla extract in a blender.
2. Blend on high speed until smooth and creamy.
3. Add ice cubes if desired and blend again until desired consistency is reached.

4. Pour into glasses and serve immediately as a refreshing and protein-packed breakfast smoothie.

Brown Rice and Veggie Breakfast Stir-Fry

Ingredients:

- 1 cup cooked brown rice
- 1/2 cup diced mixed vegetables (such as bell peppers, carrots, broccoli, and mushrooms)
- 1/4 cup diced red onion
- 1 clove garlic, minced
- 2 tablespoons olive oil
- 2 large eggs
- 2 tablespoons low-sodium soy sauce
- 1/2 teaspoon sesame oil (optional)
- Fresh green onions for garnish (optional)

Directions:

1. Heat olive oil in a skillet or wok over medium heat. Add minced garlic and sauté for 1 minute.

2. Add diced red onion and mixed vegetables to the skillet. Cook for 5-7 minutes, stirring occasionally, until the vegetables are tender.

3. Add cooked brown rice to the skillet and toss to combine. Season with low-sodium soy sauce and sesame oil (if using).

4. Create two small wells in the rice and vegetable mixture and crack an egg into each well. Cover the skillet with a lid and let the eggs cook for 3-4 minutes, or until the whites are set but the yolks are still runny.

5. Garnish with fresh green onions (if desired) and serve hot as a satisfying and fiber-rich breakfast stir-fry.

Sweet Potato and Spinach Breakfast Hash

Ingredients:

- 1 large sweet potato, peeled and diced
- 1 cup packed baby spinach leaves
- 1/2 cup diced red bell pepper

- 1/2 cup diced red onion
- 2 cloves garlic, minced
- 2 tablespoons olive oil
- Salt and pepper to taste
- 2 large eggs
- Fresh parsley for garnish (optional)

Directions:

1. Heat olive oil in a skillet over medium heat. Add minced garlic and sauté for 1 minute.
2. Add diced sweet potato, red bell pepper, and red onion to the skillet. Cook for 5-7 minutes, stirring occasionally, until the sweet potato is tender.
3. Add baby spinach leaves to the skillet and toss to combine. Cook for another 2-3 minutes, until the spinach wilts.
4. Season with salt and pepper to taste.
5. Create two small wells in the hash and crack an egg into each well. Cover the skillet with a lid and let the eggs cook for 3-4 minutes, or until the whites are set but the yolks are still runny.

6. Garnish with fresh parsley (if desired) and serve hot as a delicious and nutrient-rich breakfast hash.

Avocado and Egg Breakfast Sandwich

Ingredients:

- 2 slices whole-grain bread
- 1 ripe avocado
- 2 large eggs
- Salt and pepper to taste
- Fresh basil leaves for garnish (optional)

Directions:

1. Toast the slices of whole-grain bread to your desired level of crispiness.
2. Cut the ripe avocado in half and remove the pit. Scoop out the flesh of one avocado half and mash it with a fork in a bowl. Season with salt and pepper to taste.

3. Spread the mashed avocado onto one side of each slice of toasted bread.

4. Heat a non-stick skillet over medium heat. Crack an egg into the skillet and cook for 2-3 minutes, or until the whites are set but the yolk is still runny. Season with salt and pepper to taste.

5. Place the cooked egg on top of the mashed avocado on one slice of bread.

6. Repeat the process with the remaining egg and slice of bread.

7. Top each sandwich with fresh basil leaves (if desired) for added flavor and aroma.

8. Serve as a satisfying and protein-packed breakfast sandwich that's rich in healthy fats and fiber.

Starting your day with a healthy and gout-friendly breakfast can set the tone for the rest of your day and support your overall well-being, especially if you suffer from gout. By incorporating wholesome ingredients and making mindful choices, you can enjoy delicious breakfast recipes that are not only satisfying but also help to manage gout symptoms.

Chapter 3: Flavorful Lunch Recipes

Lunchtime is an opportunity to refuel your body and enjoy a delicious meal in the middle of a busy day. If you're looking for flavorful lunch recipes that are not only satisfying but also healthy, you've come to the right place! In this chapter, we'll explore a variety of mouthwatering lunch ideas that are perfect for those who want to indulge in delicious food while also taking care of their health. These recipes are designed to be gout-friendly, meaning they avoid high-purine ingredients that can trigger gout flare-ups, while still being packed with flavor and nutrition. So, grab your apron and let's get cooking!

Mediterranean Chickpea Salad

Ingredients:

- 1 can of chickpeas, drained and rinsed
- 1 small cucumber, diced
- 1 small red bell pepper, diced
- 1/4 red onion, finely chopped

- 1/2 cup cherry tomatoes, halved
- 1/4 cup Kalamata olives, pitted and halved
- 2 tablespoons chopped fresh parsley
- 2 tablespoons extra-virgin olive oil
- 1 tablespoon red wine vinegar
- 1 teaspoon dried oregano
- Salt and pepper to taste

Directions:

1. In a large mixing bowl, combine the chickpeas, cucumber, red bell pepper, red onion, cherry tomatoes, Kalamata olives, and chopped parsley.
2. In a small bowl, whisk together the olive oil, red wine vinegar, dried oregano, salt, and pepper to make the dressing.
3. Pour the dressing over the chickpea salad and toss gently to coat all the ingredients.
4. Serve chilled and enjoy the refreshing flavors of the Mediterranean in this delicious and satisfying salad.

Grilled Chicken and Veggie Skewers

Ingredients:

- 1 pound boneless, skinless chicken breasts, cut into chunks
- 1 small red bell pepper, cut into chunks
- 1 small green bell pepper, cut into chunks
- 1 small red onion, cut into chunks
- 1 small zucchini, cut into rounds
- 1 small yellow squash, cut into rounds
- 2 tablespoons olive oil
- 2 tablespoons freshly squeezed lemon juice
- 2 cloves garlic, minced
- 1 teaspoon dried oregano
- 1/2 teaspoon paprika
- Salt and pepper to taste

Directions:

1. In a bowl, whisk together the olive oil, lemon juice, minced garlic, dried oregano, paprika, salt, and pepper to make the marinade.

2. Thread the chicken chunks and veggies onto skewers, alternating between chicken and veggies.

3. Place the skewers in a shallow dish and pour the marinade over them, coating them evenly.

4. Cover and refrigerate for at least 30 minutes to allow the flavors to meld.

5. Preheat a grill or grill pan over medium-high heat. Grill the chicken and veggie skewers for 8-10 minutes, turning occasionally, until the chicken is cooked through and the veggies are tender.

6. Remove from the grill and let them rest for a few minutes before serving. These flavorful and juicy chicken and veggie skewers are perfect for a satisfying and protein-packed lunch.

Roasted Veggie and Quinoa Salad

Ingredients:

- 1 cup quinoa, rinsed and drained
- 2 cups water
- 1 small red bell pepper, diced
- 1 small yellow bell pepper, diced

- 1 small red onion, thinly sliced
- 1 small zucchini, diced
- 1 small yellow squash, diced
- 1 cup cherry tomatoes, halved
- 2 cloves garlic, minced
- 2 tablespoons olive oil
- 1 teaspoon dried thyme
- 1/2 teaspoon smoked paprika
- Salt and pepper to taste
- 1/4 cup chopped fresh basil

Directions:

1. Preheat the oven to 400°F (200°C) and line a baking sheet with parchment paper.

2. In a medium saucepan, combine the quinoa and water and bring to a boil. Reduce heat to low, cover, and simmer for 15-20 minutes, or until the quinoa is cooked and the water has been absorbed.

3. In a large mixing bowl, toss together the diced bell peppers, sliced red onion, diced zucchini, diced

yellow squash, minced garlic, olive oil, dried thyme, smoked paprika, salt, and pepper.

4. Spread the veggie mixture onto the prepared baking sheet and roast in the preheated oven for 20-25 minutes, stirring occasionally, until the veggies are tender and slightly caramelized.

5. In a large serving bowl, combine the roasted veggies with the cooked quinoa and toss gently to combine.

6. Garnish with chopped fresh basil before serving. This roasted veggie and quinoa salad is packed with flavor, fiber, and protein, making it a perfect option for a wholesome and filling lunch.

Tuna Salad Stuffed Avocado

Ingredients:

- 2 ripe avocados
- 1 can of tuna, drained
- 1/4 cup diced red onion
- 1/4 cup diced celery
- 1/4 cup diced cucumber
- 2 tablespoons mayonnaise

- 1 tablespoon freshly squeezed lemon juice
- 1 teaspoon Dijon mustard
- Salt and pepper to taste
- Fresh parsley for garnish

Directions:

1. Cut the avocados in half and remove the pits. Scoop out a little bit of flesh from each half to create a small well for the tuna salad.
2. In a medium mixing bowl, combine the drained tuna, diced red onion, diced celery, diced cucumber, mayonnaise, lemon juice, Dijon mustard, salt, and pepper. Stir to combine.
3. Spoon the tuna salad into the avocado halves, filling the wells generously.
4. Garnish with fresh parsley before serving. These tuna salad stuffed avocados are not only delicious but also packed with healthy fats, protein, and veggies, making them a perfect lunch option for a quick and satisfying meal.

Veggie Hummus Wrap

Ingredients:

- 4 whole wheat tortillas
- 1 cup hummus
- 1 small red bell pepper, thinly sliced
- 1 small yellow bell pepper, thinly sliced
- 1 small cucumber, thinly sliced
- 1 small carrot, grated
- 1 small red onion, thinly sliced
- 1/4 cup chopped fresh cilantro
- Salt and pepper to taste

Directions:

1. Lay out the whole wheat tortillas on a clean surface.
2. Spread about 1/4 cup of hummus on each tortilla, leaving a small border around the edges.
3. Layer the thinly sliced bell peppers, cucumber slices, grated carrot, sliced red onion, and chopped cilantro evenly over the hummus on each tortilla.
4. Sprinkle with a pinch of salt and pepper to taste.

5. Roll up the tortillas tightly, tucking in the sides as you go to create a wrap.

6. Slice the wraps in half diagonally and serve. These veggie hummus wraps are loaded with crunchy veggies and creamy hummus, making them a healthy and delicious lunch option that's easy to pack and take on the go.

Caprese Salad with Balsamic Glaze

Ingredients:

- 2 cups cherry or grape tomatoes, halved
- 8 oz fresh mozzarella cheese, cubed
- 1/4 cup chopped fresh basil
- 2 tablespoons balsamic glaze
- 2 tablespoons extra virgin olive oil
- Salt and pepper to taste

Directions:

1. In a large mixing bowl, combine the halved cherry or grape tomatoes, cubed fresh mozzarella cheese, and chopped fresh basil.

2. Drizzle with balsamic glaze and extra virgin olive oil.

3. Season with a pinch of salt and pepper to taste.

4. Toss gently to coat all the ingredients in the dressing.

5. Serve as a refreshing and flavorful Caprese salad. This classic Italian salad is a perfect lunch option for a light and refreshing meal that's bursting with the flavors of summer.

Chickpea and Vegetable Stir-Fry

Ingredients:

- 1 tablespoon vegetable oil
- 1 small red onion, thinly sliced
- 2 cloves garlic, minced
- 1 small red bell pepper, thinly sliced
- 1 small yellow bell pepper, thinly sliced
- 1 small zucchini, thinly sliced
- 1 small yellow squash, thinly sliced
- 1 cup cooked chickpeas
- 2 tablespoons soy sauce
- 1 tablespoon hoisin sauce

- 1 tablespoon rice vinegar
- 1/2 teaspoon sesame oil
- Salt and pepper to taste
- Cooked brown rice for serving

Directions:

1. In a large skillet or wok, heat the vegetable oil over medium-high heat.
2. Add the sliced red onion and minced garlic, and stir-fry for 2-3 minutes until fragrant.
3. Add the sliced red and yellow bell peppers, zucchini, and yellow squash to the skillet, and stir-fry for another 3-4 minutes until the veggies are slightly tender but still crispy.
4. Add the cooked chickpeas to the skillet, and stir-fry for another 2-3 minutes to heat them through.
5. In a small bowl, whisk together the soy sauce, hoisin sauce, rice vinegar, sesame oil, salt, and pepper.
6. Pour the sauce over the stir-fried veggies and chickpeas in the skillet, and toss gently to coat everything in the sauce.

7. Cook for another 1-2 minutes until the sauce thickens slightly.

8. Remove from heat and serve over cooked brown rice for a satisfying and flavorful lunch option that's packed with protein and veggies.

Moroccan Spiced Lentil Stew

Ingredients:

- 1 tablespoon olive oil
- 1 small red onion, finely diced
- 2 cloves garlic, minced
- 1 small carrot, peeled and diced
- 1 small zucchini, diced
- 1 small yellow squash, diced
- 1 teaspoon ground cumin
- 1/2 teaspoon ground turmeric
- 1/2 teaspoon ground cinnamon
- 1/4 teaspoon ground ginger
- 1/4 teaspoon ground paprika
- 1/4 teaspoon cayenne pepper (optional)
- 1 cup dried green or brown lentils, rinsed and drained

- 4 cups vegetable broth
- 1 can diced tomatoes
- Salt and pepper to taste
- Fresh cilantro for garnish
- Cooked couscous for serving

Directions:

1. In a large pot, heat the olive oil over medium heat.
2. Add the diced red onion and minced garlic, and sauté for 2-3 minutes until softened.
3. Add the diced carrot, zucchini, and yellow squash to the pot, and sauté for another 3-4 minutes until the veggies start to soften.
4. Stir in the ground cumin, turmeric, cinnamon, ginger, paprika, and cayenne pepper (if using), and cook for another 1-2 minutes until fragrant.
5. Add the rinsed and drained lentils, vegetable broth, and diced tomatoes to the pot.
6. Bring the mixture to a boil, then reduce the heat to low, cover the pot, and simmer for 25-30 minutes until the lentils are tender.

7. Season with salt and pepper to taste.

8. Serve the Moroccan spiced lentil stew hot, garnished with fresh cilantro, and accompanied by cooked couscous for a hearty and flavorful lunch option that's rich in plant-based protein and warming spices.

Greek Veggie Wrap with Tzatziki Sauce

Ingredients for the Tzatziki Sauce:

- 1 cup plain Greek yogurt
- 1/2 small cucumber, grated and squeezed to remove excess moisture
- 1 clove garlic, minced
- 1 tablespoon fresh lemon juice
- 1 tablespoon extra virgin olive oil
- 1 tablespoon chopped fresh dill (or 1 teaspoon dried dill)
- Salt and pepper to taste

Ingredients for the Greek Veggie Wrap:

- 4 large whole wheat wraps or tortillas
- 1 small red onion, thinly sliced
- 1 small cucumber, thinly sliced
- 1 small red bell pepper, thinly sliced
- 1 small yellow bell pepper, thinly sliced
- 1 small zucchini, thinly sliced
- 1 small yellow squash, thinly sliced
- 1/2 cup crumbled feta cheese
- Fresh spinach leaves

Directions for the Tzatziki Sauce:

1. In a medium mixing bowl, combine the Greek yogurt, grated cucumber, minced garlic, lemon juice, olive oil, chopped fresh dill, salt, and pepper.
2. Stir well to combine, and refrigerate for at least 30 minutes to allow the flavors to meld together.

Directions for the Greek Veggie Wrap:

1. Lay out the whole wheat wraps or tortillas on a clean surface.

2. Spread a generous amount of the prepared Tzatziki sauce onto each wrap.

3. Layer the thinly sliced red onion, cucumber, red and yellow bell peppers, zucchini, yellow squash, crumbled feta cheese, and fresh spinach leaves onto each wrap.

4. Roll up the wraps tightly, tucking in the sides as you go.

5. Cut the wraps in half or into smaller pinwheels for a convenient and delicious lunch option that's filled with the flavors of the Mediterranean.

Chapter 4: Wholesome Dinner Recipes

Dinner time is a special part of the day when families and friends come together to share a meal and create cherished memories. It's also an opportunity to nourish our bodies with wholesome, nutritious food that fuels us for the next day. If you're looking for delicious and healthy dinner recipes that are easy to prepare, look no further! In this chapter, we will explore a variety of wholesome dinner recipes that are perfect for any occasion, from weeknight dinners to special gatherings. Packed with flavorful ingredients and simple cooking techniques, these recipes will help you create a satisfying meal that is both nutritious and tasty.

Lemon Garlic Baked Salmon

Ingredients:

- 4 salmon fillets
- 4 cloves garlic, minced
- 1 lemon, zested and juiced

- 2 tablespoons olive oil
- Salt and pepper, to taste
- Fresh parsley, for garnish

Directions:

1. Preheat your oven to 400°F (200°C) and line a baking sheet with parchment paper.
2. In a small bowl, mix together minced garlic, lemon zest, lemon juice, olive oil, salt, and pepper to form a marinade.
3. Place the salmon fillets on the prepared baking sheet and brush the marinade over the top of each fillet.
4. Bake the salmon in the preheated oven for 12-15 minutes, or until the fish is cooked through and flakes easily with a fork.
5. Remove from the oven and let the salmon rest for a few minutes before serving.
6. Garnish with fresh parsley and serve with your favorite side dish, such as roasted vegetables or quinoa, for a complete and wholesome dinner.

Spicy Shrimp and Veggie Stir-Fry

Ingredients:

- 1 pound large shrimp, peeled and deveined
- 2 cloves garlic, minced
- 1 inch fresh ginger, minced
- 1 tablespoon vegetable oil
- 1 red bell pepper, thinly sliced
- 1 yellow bell pepper, thinly sliced
- 1 cup snow peas
- 1/4 cup low-sodium soy sauce
- 2 tablespoons hoisin sauce
- 1 tablespoon Sriracha sauce (adjust to taste)
- 1 tablespoon cornstarch
- Green onions, sliced, for garnish

Directions:

1. In a small bowl, whisk together soy sauce, hoisin sauce, Sriracha sauce, and cornstarch to create a sauce. Set aside.

2. Heat vegetable oil in a large skillet or wok over medium-high heat.

3. Add minced garlic and ginger to the hot oil and sauté for 1-2 minutes until fragrant.

4. Add the shrimp to the skillet and cook for 2-3 minutes per side until pink and cooked through. Remove the shrimp from the skillet and set aside.

5. In the same skillet, add more oil if needed, and then add the sliced bell peppers and snow peas. Stir-fry for 2-3 minutes until the vegetables are crisp-tender.

6. Add the cooked shrimp back to the skillet with the vegetables, and then pour in the sauce. Stir-fry for an additional 2-3 minutes, or until the sauce has thickened and coated the shrimp and vegetables.

7. Remove from heat and garnish with sliced green onions.

8. Serve the spicy shrimp and veggie stir-fry over steamed brown rice or whole wheat noodles for a wholesome and satisfying dinner.

Herb-Roasted Chicken with Steamed Veggies

Ingredients:

- 4 bone-in, skin-on chicken thighs
- 2 tablespoons olive oil
- 1 tablespoon fresh rosemary, minced
- 1 tablespoon fresh thyme, minced
- 1 tablespoon fresh parsley, minced
- Salt and pepper, to taste
- 1 pound mixed vegetables (such as carrots, broccoli, and cauliflower), washed and trimmed

Directions:

1. Preheat your oven to 425°F (220°C) and line a baking sheet with parchment paper.
2. Pat dry the chicken thighs with a paper towel and place them on the prepared baking sheet.
3. In a small bowl, mix together the minced rosemary, thyme, parsley, olive oil, salt, and pepper to create a herb rub.

4. Rub the herb mixture evenly over the chicken thighs, making sure to coat all sides.

5. Roast the chicken in the preheated oven for 25-30 minutes, or until the internal temperature reaches 165°F (75°C) and the skin is golden and crispy.

6. While the chicken is roasting, prepare the steamed vegetables by placing them in a steamer basket over a pot of boiling water. Steam for 5-7 minutes, or until the vegetables are tender but still slightly crisp.

7. Remove the chicken from the oven and let it rest for a few minutes before serving.

8. Serve the herb-roasted chicken with steamed veggies for a wholesome and satisfying dinner. Optionally, you can also serve it with a side of quinoa or roasted potatoes for a more filling meal.

Vegetarian Lentil and Vegetable Stew

Ingredients:

- 1 tablespoon olive oil
- 1 onion, diced

- 2 carrots, peeled and diced
- 2 celery stalks, diced
- 3 cloves garlic, minced
- 1 teaspoon smoked paprika
- 1/2 teaspoon cumin
- 1/2 teaspoon turmeric
- 1/4 teaspoon cinnamon
- 1 cup dried green or brown lentils, rinsed and drained
- 1 can (14 ounces) diced tomatoes
- 4 cups vegetable broth
- 2 bay leaves
- Salt and pepper, to taste
- Fresh parsley, for garnish

Directions:

1. Heat olive oil in a large pot over medium heat.
2. Add diced onion, carrots, and celery to the pot and sauté for 5-7 minutes, or until the vegetables are softened.

3. Add minced garlic, smoked paprika, cumin, turmeric, and cinnamon to the pot and cook for another 1-2 minutes until fragrant.

4. Add lentils, diced tomatoes, vegetable broth, bay leaves, salt, and pepper to the pot. Stir well to combine.

5. Bring the stew to a boil, then reduce the heat to low and let it simmer for 25-30 minutes, or until the lentils are tender.

6. Remove the bay leaves from the stew and discard.

7. Taste and adjust the seasoning with salt and pepper, if needed.

8. Serve the vegetarian lentil and vegetable stew hot, garnished with fresh parsley for a wholesome and hearty dinner. You can also serve it with a slice of crusty whole grain bread or a side of steamed greens for a complete meal.

Baked Sweet Potato and Black Bean Enchiladas

Ingredients:

- 2 large sweet potatoes, peeled and diced
- 1 tablespoon olive oil
- 1 onion, diced
- 3 cloves garlic, minced
- 1 can (15 ounces) black beans, rinsed and drained
- 1 can (10 ounces) enchilada sauce
- 1 teaspoon chili powder
- 1/2 teaspoon cumin
- Salt and pepper, to taste
- 8 whole grain tortillas
- 1 cup shredded cheddar or Mexican blend cheese
- Chopped fresh cilantro, for garnish

Directions:

1. Preheat your oven to 375°F (190°C) and grease a 9x13-inch baking dish.

2. Place the diced sweet potatoes on a baking sheet, drizzle with olive oil, and toss to coat. Roast in the preheated oven for 20-25 minutes, or until the sweet potatoes are tender and lightly golden.

3. In a large skillet, heat olive oil over medium heat. Add diced onion and minced garlic to the skillet and sauté for 5-7 minutes, or until the onion is softened.

4. Add the black beans, enchilada sauce, chili powder, cumin, salt, and pepper to the skillet. Stir well to combine and let the mixture simmer for 5-7 minutes, or until heated through.

5. Once the sweet potatoes are roasted, add them to the skillet with the black bean mixture and stir gently to combine.

6. Warm the tortillas according to package instructions to make them pliable.

7. Spoon a generous amount of the sweet potato and black bean mixture onto each tortilla, roll it up tightly, and place it seam-side down in the prepared baking dish.

8. Repeat with the remaining tortillas and filling until all the enchiladas are assembled in the baking dish.

9. Sprinkle shredded cheese evenly over the top of the enchiladas.

10. Bake in the preheated oven for 20-25 minutes, or until the cheese is melted and bubbly.

11. Remove from the oven and let the enchiladas cool for a few minutes before serving.

12. Garnish with chopped cilantro for a burst of fresh flavor and serve the baked sweet potato and black bean enchiladas with a side of Mexican rice or a simple green salad for a wholesome and satisfying dinner.

Grilled Salmon with Lemon-Dill Sauce

Ingredients:

- 4 salmon fillets (6 ounces each)
- 2 tablespoons olive oil
- 2 tablespoons freshly squeezed lemon juice
- 2 tablespoons chopped fresh dill
- 2 cloves garlic, minced
- Salt and pepper, to taste

- Lemon slices, for garnish

For Lemon-Dill Sauce:

- 1/2 cup Greek yogurt
- 1 tablespoon freshly squeezed lemon juice
- 1 tablespoon chopped fresh dill
- 1 clove garlic, minced
- Salt and pepper, to taste

Directions:

1. Preheat your grill to medium-high heat.
2. In a small bowl, whisk together olive oil, lemon juice, chopped dill, minced garlic, salt, and pepper to create a marinade for the salmon.
3. Place the salmon fillets in a shallow dish and pour the marinade over them, making sure to coat all sides.
4. Let the salmon marinate for 15-20 minutes to allow the flavors to meld.

5. Meanwhile, in another small bowl, mix together Greek yogurt, lemon juice, chopped dill, minced garlic, salt, and pepper to make the lemon-dill sauce. Stir well to combine.

6. After marinating, remove the salmon fillets from the marinade and grill them on medium-high heat for 3-4 minutes per side, or until they are cooked to your desired level of doneness.

7. Transfer the grilled salmon to a serving plate and let it rest for a few minutes.

8. Serve the grilled salmon hot, garnished with lemon slices and a dollop of lemon-dill sauce on top.

9. Pair it with a side of roasted vegetables or quinoa for a wholesome and nutritious dinner.

Veggie Stir-Fry with Brown Rice

Ingredients:

- 2 cups cooked brown rice
- 2 tablespoons vegetable oil
- 1 small red onion, thinly sliced
- 2 cloves garlic, minced

- 1 cup sliced bell peppers (any color)
- 1 cup sliced carrots
- 1 cup sliced mushrooms
- 1 cup broccoli florets
- 1 cup snap peas
- 1/4 cup low-sodium soy sauce
- 2 tablespoons hoisin sauce
- 1 tablespoon rice vinegar
- 1 tablespoon cornstarch
- 1/2 cup vegetable broth
- Salt and pepper, to taste
- Sesame seeds, for garnish
- Chopped green onions, for garnish

Directions:

1. Heat vegetable oil in a large skillet or wok over medium-high heat.
2. Add sliced red onion and minced garlic to the skillet and sauté for 2-3 minutes, or until fragrant.

3. Add sliced bell peppers, carrots, mushrooms, broccoli florets, and snap peas to the skillet. Stir-fry for 4-5 minutes, or until the vegetables are crisp-tender.

4. In a small bowl, whisk together soy sauce, hoisin sauce, rice vinegar, cornstarch, and vegetable broth to make the stir-fry sauce.

5. Pour the sauce over the vegetables in the skillet and toss to coat evenly. Cook for another 2-3 minutes, or until the sauce has thickened.

6. Season with salt and pepper to taste.

7. Add the cooked brown rice to the skillet and stir-fry for an additional 2-3 minutes, or until the rice is heated through and well combined with the vegetables and sauce.

8. Remove from heat and garnish with sesame seeds and chopped green onions for added flavor and presentation.

9. Serve the veggie stir-fry with brown rice as a wholesome and satisfying dinner option.

Wholesome dinner recipes are a fantastic way to nourish your body and enjoy delicious meals that are both satisfying and nutritious. From hearty soups and stews to flavorful stir-fries, roasted chicken, stuffed bell peppers, and baked salmon with roasted vegetables, there are endless options to choose from when it comes to wholesome dinner ideas.

Chapter 5: Nutrient-Rich Side Dishes

Side dishes are often overlooked, but they can be the star of any meal. They add depth, flavor, and nutrition to your plate, making your meal truly satisfying and wholesome. When it comes to side dishes, opting for nutrient-rich ingredients is key to ensure you're getting the most out of your meal. In this chapter, we'll explore some delicious and wholesome side dish recipes that are packed with nutrients to elevate your meals to a whole new level of taste and health.

Roasted Garlic and Herb Cauliflower

Ingredients:

- 1 head of cauliflower, cut into florets
- 4 cloves of garlic, minced
- 2 tbsp olive oil
- 1 tbsp chopped fresh herbs (such as rosemary, thyme, or parsley)
- Salt and pepper to taste

Directions:

1. Preheat your oven to 400°F (200°C) and line a baking sheet with parchment paper.
2. In a large bowl, toss the cauliflower florets with minced garlic, olive oil, chopped fresh herbs, salt, and pepper until evenly coated.
3. Spread the cauliflower in a single layer on the prepared baking sheet.
4. Roast in the preheated oven for 20-25 minutes, or until the cauliflower is tender and golden brown, tossing occasionally to ensure even cooking.
5. Remove from the oven and serve hot as a flavorful and nutrient-rich side dish.

Ginger Sesame Broccoli

Ingredients:

- 1 lb broccoli florets
- 2 tbsp sesame oil
- 1 tbsp soy sauce
- 1 tbsp freshly grated ginger

- 2 cloves of garlic, minced
- 1 tbsp sesame seeds
- Salt and pepper to taste

Directions:

1. Steam the broccoli florets until they are crisp-tender, about 3-4 minutes. Drain and set aside.
2. In a small bowl, whisk together sesame oil, soy sauce, freshly grated ginger, minced garlic, sesame seeds, salt, and pepper to create a dressing.
3. In a large skillet, heat the dressing over medium heat.
4. Add the steamed broccoli to the skillet and toss to coat the florets evenly with the dressing.
5. Cook for an additional 2-3 minutes, stirring occasionally, until the broccoli is heated through and the flavors have melded.
6. Serve hot as a delicious and nutrient-rich side dish that's bursting with Asian-inspired flavors.

Balsamic Glazed Brussels Sprouts

Ingredients:

- 1 lb Brussels sprouts, trimmed and halved
- 2 tbsp balsamic vinegar
- 2 tbsp olive oil
- 1 tbsp honey
- Salt and pepper to taste

Directions:

1. Preheat your oven to 400°F (200°C) and line a baking sheet with parchment paper.
2. In a large bowl, whisk together balsamic vinegar, olive oil, honey, salt, and pepper to create a glaze.
3. Add the halved Brussels sprouts to the bowl and toss to coat them evenly with the glaze.
4. Spread the Brussels sprouts in a single layer on the prepared baking sheet.
5. Roast in the preheated oven for 20-25 minutes, or until the Brussels sprouts are caramelized and tender, tossing occasionally to ensure even cooking.

6. Remove from the oven and serve hot as a tangy and flavorful side dish that's loaded with nutrients.

Lemon-Parsley Quinoa

Ingredients:

- 1 cup quinoa, rinsed and drained
- 2 cups vegetable broth or water
- 2 tbsp freshly squeezed lemon juice
- 2 tbsp chopped fresh parsley
- 2 tbsp olive oil
- 2 cloves of garlic, minced
- Salt and pepper to taste

Directions:

1. In a medium saucepan, combine quinoa and vegetable broth or water. Bring to a boil over high heat.
2. Reduce heat to low, cover, and simmer for 15-20 minutes, or until quinoa is cooked and liquid is absorbed.

3. Remove from heat and let quinoa cool slightly.

4. In a large bowl, whisk together lemon juice, chopped fresh parsley, olive oil, minced garlic, salt, and pepper to create a dressing.

5. Add the cooked quinoa to the bowl and toss to coat the quinoa evenly with the dressing.

6. Serve warm or chilled as a refreshing and protein-packed side dish that's bursting with zesty flavors.

Spinach and Mushroom Sauté

Ingredients:

- 2 tbsp butter or olive oil
- 8 oz fresh mushrooms, sliced
- 2 cloves of garlic, minced
- 1 lb fresh spinach leaves
- Salt and pepper to taste
- Grated Parmesan cheese for garnish (optional)

Directions:

1. In a large skillet, melt butter or heat olive oil over medium heat.

2. Add sliced mushrooms to the skillet and sauté for 4-5 minutes, or until mushrooms are golden brown and tender.

3. Add minced garlic to the skillet and sauté for an additional 1 minute.

4. Add fresh spinach leaves to the skillet, in batches if necessary, and cook until wilted, stirring occasionally.

5. Season with salt and pepper to taste.

6. Remove from heat and sprinkle with grated Parmesan cheese, if desired, for an extra burst of flavor.

7. Serve hot as a nutrient-rich and flavorful side dish that's packed with vitamins and minerals.

Oven-Roasted Sweet Potato Wedges

Ingredients:

- 2 large sweet potatoes, peeled and cut into wedges
- 2 tbsp olive oil
- 1 tsp paprika
- 1/2 tsp garlic powder

- 1/2 tsp onion powder
- 1/2 tsp dried thyme
- Salt and pepper to taste

Directions:

1. Preheat your oven to 425°F (220°C) and line a baking sheet with parchment paper.
2. In a large bowl, toss sweet potato wedges with olive oil, paprika, garlic powder, onion powder, dried thyme, salt, and pepper until evenly coated.
3. Spread the sweet potato wedges in a single layer on the prepared baking sheet.
4. Roast in the preheated oven for 20-25 minutes, or until the sweet potatoes are tender and crispy, flipping halfway through to ensure even cooking.
5. Remove from the oven and serve hot as a delectable and nutrient-rich side dish that's loaded with natural sweetness and warmth.

Quinoa and Vegetable Stir-Fry

Ingredients:

- 1 cup quinoa, rinsed and drained
- 2 cups vegetable broth or water
- 2 tbsp olive oil
- 1 small red bell pepper, thinly sliced
- 1 small yellow bell pepper, thinly sliced
- 1 small zucchini, halved and thinly sliced
- 1 small carrot, peeled and julienned
- 2 cloves of garlic, minced
- 2 tbsp soy sauce
- 1 tbsp rice vinegar
- 1/2 tsp sesame oil
- Salt and pepper to taste
- Chopped green onions for garnish (optional)

Directions:

1. In a medium saucepan, combine quinoa and vegetable broth or water. Bring to a boil over high heat.

2. Reduce heat to low, cover, and simmer for 15-20 minutes, or until quinoa is cooked and liquid is absorbed.

3. In a large skillet or wok, heat olive oil over medium-high heat.

4. Add sliced red and yellow bell peppers, zucchini, and julienned carrot to the skillet, and stir-fry for 3-4 minutes, or until the vegetables are crisp-tender.

5. Add minced garlic to the skillet and stir-fry for an additional 1 minute.

6. Stir in cooked quinoa, soy sauce, rice vinegar, sesame oil, salt, and pepper, and continue to stir-fry for 2-3 minutes, or until the flavors are well combined and the quinoa is heated through.

7. Remove from heat and garnish with chopped green onions, if desired.

8. Serve hot as a nutritious and colorful side dish that's packed with protein, fiber, and an array of delicious vegetables.

Roasted Brussels Sprouts with Balsamic Glaze

Ingredients:

- 1 lb Brussels sprouts, trimmed and halved
- 2 tbsp olive oil
- Salt and pepper to taste
- 1/4 cup balsamic vinegar
- 2 tbsp honey or maple syrup

Directions:

1. Preheat your oven to 400°F (200°C) and line a baking sheet with parchment paper.
2. In a large bowl, toss Brussels sprouts with olive oil, salt, and pepper until evenly coated.
3. Spread the Brussels sprouts in a single layer on the prepared baking sheet.
4. Roast in the preheated oven for 20-25 minutes, or until the Brussels sprouts are tender and lightly charred, flipping halfway through to ensure even cooking.

5. In a small saucepan, combine balsamic vinegar and honey or maple syrup. Bring to a simmer over medium heat, then reduce heat to low and simmer for 5-7 minutes, or until the mixture has thickened into a glaze-like consistency.

6. Remove the roasted Brussels sprouts from the oven and drizzle with the balsamic glaze.

7. Toss gently to coat the Brussels sprouts with the glaze.

8. Serve hot as a delectable and nutrient-rich side dish that's bursting with caramelized flavors and tangy sweetness.

Nutrient-rich side dishes are a delicious and healthy way to enhance your meals and provide your body with essential vitamins, minerals, fiber, and other nutrients. They can add color, texture, and flavor to your plate, making your meals more satisfying and enjoyable.

Chapter 6: Scrumptious Snack Recipes

When it comes to snacking, it's all about finding the perfect balance between deliciousness and healthiness. Snacks can be a great way to curb hunger between meals, satisfy cravings, and keep your energy levels up throughout the day. And if you're someone who suffers from gout or is trying to manage uric acid levels, finding gout-friendly snack options becomes even more important. But fear not, because in this chapter, we'll delve into some mouthwatering snack recipes that are not only packed with flavor, but also gout-friendly, so you can indulge guilt-free!

Greek Hummus with Fresh Veggies

Ingredients:

- 1 can chickpeas, drained and rinsed
- 2 cloves garlic, minced
- 2 tablespoons tahini
- 2 tablespoons extra-virgin olive oil

- 1 tablespoon freshly squeezed lemon juice
- 1/2 teaspoon ground cumin
- 1/4 teaspoon paprika
- Salt and black pepper to taste
- Assorted fresh veggies for dipping (carrots, cucumbers, bell peppers, cherry tomatoes, etc.)

Directions:

1. In a food processor, combine the chickpeas, minced garlic, tahini, olive oil, lemon juice, cumin, paprika, salt, and pepper. Process until smooth and creamy, scraping down the sides of the bowl as needed.
2. Taste and adjust seasoning if desired. If the hummus is too thick, you can add a little more olive oil or lemon juice to achieve your desired consistency.
3. Transfer the hummus to a serving bowl and serve with an assortment of fresh veggies for dipping. Enjoy!

Spicy Edamame

Ingredients:

- 1 cup frozen edamame
- 1 tablespoon sesame oil
- 1 tablespoon soy sauce
- 1/2 teaspoon sriracha sauce (or more to taste)
- 1/2 teaspoon grated ginger
- 1/2 teaspoon sesame seeds (optional)

Directions:

1. Cook the frozen edamame according to package instructions. Drain and set aside.
2. In a small bowl, whisk together the sesame oil, soy sauce, sriracha sauce, grated ginger, and sesame seeds (if using).
3. Add the cooked edamame to the bowl with the sauce and toss until well-coated.
4. Transfer the spicy edamame to a serving plate and serve warm. Enjoy the fiery kick of this tasty snack!

Roasted Chickpeas with Turmeric and Cumin

Ingredients:

- 1 can chickpeas, drained and rinsed
- 1 tablespoon extra-virgin olive oil
- 1 teaspoon ground turmeric
- 1/2 teaspoon ground cumin
- 1/2 teaspoon paprika
- 1/4 teaspoon cayenne pepper (optional)
- Salt to taste

Directions:

1. Preheat your oven to 400°F (200°C) and line a baking sheet with parchment paper.
2. In a bowl, toss the chickpeas with olive oil, ground turmeric, ground cumin, paprika, cayenne pepper (if using), and salt until well-coated.
3. Spread the chickpeas in a single layer on the prepared baking sheet.

4. Roast in the preheated oven for 25-30 minutes, or until the chickpeas are golden and crispy, stirring occasionally to ensure even cooking.

5. Remove from the oven and let cool slightly before serving. Enjoy the crunchy, flavorful goodness of these roasted chickpeas!

Cheesy Zucchini Chips

Ingredients:

- 2 small zucchini, thinly sliced
- 1/2 cup grated Parmesan cheese
- 1/2 teaspoon garlic powder
- 1/2 teaspoon onion powder
- 1/2 teaspoon dried oregano
- 1/2 teaspoon dried basil
- Salt and black pepper to taste

Directions:

1. Preheat your oven to 425°F (220°C) and line a baking sheet with parchment paper.

2. In a bowl, combine the grated Parmesan cheese, garlic powder, onion powder, dried oregano, dried basil, salt, and pepper. Mix well.

3. Dip each zucchini slice into the Parmesan cheese mixture, pressing lightly to adhere the cheese to the slice.

4. Place the coated zucchini slices in a single layer on the prepared baking sheet.

5. Bake in the preheated oven for 10-12 minutes, or until the edges are crispy and golden brown.

6. Remove from the oven and let cool for a few minutes before serving. Enjoy the irresistible combination of cheesy and crispy zucchini chips!

Guacamole with Veggie Sticks

Ingredients:

- 2 ripe avocados, peeled and pitted
- 1 small red onion, finely chopped
- 1 small jalapeno, seeds and ribs removed, finely chopped
- 1 clove garlic, minced

- 1 tablespoon freshly squeezed lime juice
- 1/2 teaspoon ground cumin
- Salt and black pepper to taste
- Assorted veggie sticks for dipping (carrots, celery, bell peppers, etc.)

Directions:

1. In a bowl, mash the avocados with a fork or a potato masher until smooth but still slightly chunky.
2. Add the chopped red onion, jalapeno, minced garlic, lime juice, ground cumin, salt, and pepper to the bowl. Mix well.
3. Taste and adjust seasoning if desired. Add more lime juice or salt to taste.
4. Transfer the guacamole to a serving bowl and serve with an assortment of veggie sticks for dipping. Enjoy the creamy and tangy goodness of homemade guacamole!

Greek Yogurt with Berries and Nuts

Ingredients:

- 1 cup plain Greek yogurt
- 1 cup mixed berries (strawberries, blueberries, raspberries, etc.)
- 1/4 cup chopped nuts (almonds, walnuts, pistachios, etc.)
- 1 tablespoon honey (optional)

Directions:

1. In a bowl, spoon the Greek yogurt.
2. Top with mixed berries and chopped nuts.
3. Drizzle with honey if desired for added sweetness.
4. Mix everything together gently with a spoon and enjoy the protein-packed, nutrient-rich goodness of this simple and satisfying snack!

Caprese Salad Skewers

Ingredients:

- Cherry tomatoes
- Fresh basil leaves
- Fresh mozzarella balls
- Balsamic glaze for drizzling

Directions:

1. On small skewers or toothpicks, thread a cherry tomato, a fresh basil leaf, and a fresh mozzarella ball.
2. Repeat with the remaining ingredients.
3. Arrange the caprese salad skewers on a serving platter.
4. Drizzle with balsamic glaze just before serving for a burst of tangy flavor.
5. Enjoy the colorful and flavorful combination of tomatoes, basil, and mozzarella in these bite-sized delights!

Snacking doesn't have to be boring or unhealthy, even if you're watching your uric acid levels due to gout. With these scrumptious snack recipes, you can indulge in deliciousness while keeping your health in mind.

Chapter 7: Delectable Dessert Recipes

Desserts are the perfect ending to any meal, and they can be a delightful treat to indulge in. However, for those who are managing health conditions such as gout, it's important to choose desserts that are not only delicious but also gout-friendly. Gout is a type of arthritis caused by the buildup of uric acid crystals in the joints, leading to severe pain and inflammation. Diet plays a crucial role in managing gout, and making smart choices when it comes to desserts can help prevent flare-ups and promote overall health. In this chapter, we will explore a variety of delectable dessert recipes that are not only tempting but also suitable for those with gout. From fruity treats to creamy delights, we have something for everyone to enjoy guilt-free.

Mixed Berry Crumble

Ingredients:

- 2 cups mixed berries (such as strawberries, blueberries, raspberries)

- 1/4 cup granulated sugar
- 1 tablespoon lemon juice
- 1/2 teaspoon vanilla extract
- 1/2 cup all-purpose flour
- 1/2 cup rolled oats
- 1/4 cup brown sugar
- 1/4 cup chopped nuts (such as almonds or walnuts)
- 1/4 cup unsalted butter, melted

Directions:

1. Preheat your oven to 375°F (190°C) and grease a baking dish.
2. In a bowl, toss the mixed berries with granulated sugar, lemon juice, and vanilla extract. Spread the berry mixture evenly in the prepared baking dish.
3. In another bowl, combine the flour, oats, brown sugar, chopped nuts, and melted butter. Stir until the mixture resembles coarse crumbs.
4. Sprinkle the crumble mixture evenly over the berry mixture in the baking dish.

5. Bake for 25-30 minutes, or until the top is golden brown and the berry mixture is bubbling.

6. Remove from the oven and let cool for a few minutes before serving. Serve warm, and enjoy the juicy and tangy sweetness of the mixed berry crumble.

Chocolate Avocado Mousse

Ingredients:

- 2 ripe avocados, peeled and pitted
- 1/4 cup unsweetened cocoa powder
- 1/4 cup pure maple syrup or honey
- 1 teaspoon vanilla extract
- A pinch of salt
- Fresh berries or chopped nuts for garnish (optional)

Directions:

1. Place the peeled and pitted avocados in a blender or food processor.

2. Add the cocoa powder, maple syrup or honey, vanilla extract, and a pinch of salt to the blender or food processor.

3. Blend or process on high speed until the mixture is smooth and creamy.

4. Taste and adjust sweetness with more maple syrup or honey, if desired.

5. Spoon the chocolate avocado mousse into individual serving dishes or ramekins.

6. Chill in the refrigerator for at least 1 hour to allow the mousse to firm up.

7. Garnish with fresh berries or chopped nuts, if desired, and serve chilled. Enjoy the rich and luscious flavor of this creamy chocolate treat.

Coconut Milk and Berry Popsicles

Ingredients:

- 1 cup mixed berries (such as strawberries, blueberries, raspberries)
- 1/4 cup pure maple syrup or honey
- 1 can (14 ounces) coconut milk

- 1 teaspoon vanilla extract

Directions:

1. In a blender, combine the mixed berries, maple syrup or honey, coconut milk, and vanilla extract.
2. Blend on high speed until the mixture is smooth and well combined.
3. Pour the berry mixture into popsicle molds, leaving a little space at the top for expansion.
4. Insert popsicle sticks into the molds and freeze for at least 4-6 hours, or until the popsicles are completely frozen.
5. Once frozen, remove the popsicles from the molds by running them under warm water for a few seconds or placing them in warm water for a minute to loosen them.
6. Serve and enjoy these refreshing and creamy coconut milk and berry popsicles on a hot summer day.

Lemon Greek Yogurt Cake

Ingredients:

- 1 1/2 cups all-purpose flour
- 1/2 cup granulated sugar
- 1/2 cup Greek yogurt
- 1/4 cup unsalted butter, melted
- 2 eggs
- 1 tablespoon lemon zest
- 2 tablespoons lemon juice
- 1 teaspoon vanilla extract
- 1/2 teaspoon baking powder
- 1/4 teaspoon baking soda
- 1/4 teaspoon salt

Directions:

1. Preheat your oven to 350°F (175°C) and grease a 9-inch round cake pan.
2. In a large bowl, whisk together the flour, sugar, baking powder, baking soda, and salt.

3. In another bowl, whisk together the Greek yogurt, melted butter, eggs, lemon zest, lemon juice, and vanilla extract.

4. Pour the wet ingredients into the dry ingredients and stir until just combined.

5. Pour the batter into the prepared cake pan and smooth the top with a spatula.

6. Bake for 25-30 minutes, or until a toothpick inserted into the center of the cake comes out clean.

7. Remove from the oven and let the cake cool in the pan for 10 minutes before transferring to a wire rack to cool completely.

8. Once cooled, you can dust the cake with powdered sugar or drizzle with a lemon glaze for added sweetness, if desired.

9. Slice and serve this tangy and moist Lemon Greek Yogurt Cake for a delightful dessert or afternoon tea treat.

Apple Walnut Crisp

Ingredients:

- 4 cups peeled and thinly sliced apples (such as Granny Smith or Honeycrisp)
- 1/2 cup all-purpose flour
- 1/2 cup rolled oats
- 1/2 cup chopped walnuts
- 1/2 cup packed brown sugar
- 1/4 cup unsalted butter, melted
- 1 teaspoon cinnamon
- 1/4 teaspoon nutmeg
- A pinch of salt

Directions:

1. Preheat your oven to 375°F (190°C) and grease a baking dish.
2. In a large bowl, combine the sliced apples, flour, rolled oats, chopped walnuts, brown sugar, melted butter, cinnamon, nutmeg, and a pinch of salt. Stir until the apple mixture is well coated.

3. Transfer the apple mixture to the prepared baking dish and spread it out evenly.

4. Bake for 30-35 minutes, or until the apples are tender and the top is golden brown and crispy.

5. Remove from the oven and let cool for a few minutes before serving.

6. Serve warm, and enjoy the comforting flavors of the soft and sweet apples paired with the crunchy walnut crumble.

Indulging in delicious desserts doesn't have to be off-limits when you're managing gout. With these delectable dessert recipes, you can satisfy your sweet tooth while making smart choices for your health. From fruity delights to creamy treats, these recipes are packed with flavor and nutrition, making them suitable for those with gout or anyone who wants to enjoy desserts in a healthier way.

Chapter 8: Beverages for Gout Management

In this chapter, we will focus on beverages that can help manage gout by incorporating gout-friendly ingredients that are known for their anti-inflammatory properties, antioxidants, and other health benefits. These delicious beverages can be a refreshing addition to your gout management plan and can help you stay hydrated while enjoying flavorful and beneficial drinks.

Cherry Juice Smoothie

Cherries are known for their potential anti-inflammatory properties and have been shown to help reduce gout flare-ups. This cherry juice smoothie is a delicious and refreshing way to incorporate cherries into your diet and manage gout.

Ingredients:

- 1 cup frozen cherries
- 1 cup almond milk

- 1 ripe banana
- 1 tablespoon honey
- 1/2 teaspoon vanilla extract
- Ice (optional)

Directions:

1. Add the frozen cherries, almond milk, ripe banana, honey, and vanilla extract to a blender.
2. Blend on high until smooth and creamy.
3. If desired, add ice for a colder and thicker smoothie.
4. Pour into glasses and serve immediately.

Cucumber and Mint Infused Water

Staying hydrated is crucial for managing gout, as it helps to flush out excess uric acid from the body. This cucumber and mint infused water is a refreshing and flavorful way to increase your water intake and keep your body hydrated.

Ingredients:

- 1/2 cucumber, thinly sliced

- 1 small handful of fresh mint leaves
- 8 cups of water
- Ice cubes

Directions:

1. In a pitcher, combine the cucumber slices and fresh mint leaves.
2. Pour the water over the cucumber and mint, and stir gently.
3. Place the pitcher in the refrigerator for at least 1 hour to allow the flavors to infuse.
4. When ready to serve, fill glasses with ice cubes and pour the infused water over the ice.
5. Stir gently and enjoy the refreshing taste of cucumber and mint in your water.

Ginger-Turmeric Tea

Ginger and turmeric are both known for their anti-inflammatory properties, and incorporating them into a warm beverage can be soothing and beneficial for managing gout. This ginger-turmeric tea is easy to make and can be enjoyed as a comforting drink throughout the day.

Ingredients:

- 1 inch fresh ginger, peeled and grated
- 1 inch fresh turmeric, peeled and grated (or 1 teaspoon ground turmeric)
- 4 cups of water
- 1 tablespoon honey (optional)
- Lemon slices (optional)

Directions:

1. In a saucepan, bring the water to a boil.
2. Add the grated ginger and turmeric (or ground turmeric) to the boiling water.
3. Reduce the heat to low and let the mixture simmer for about 10 minutes.
4. Remove the saucepan from the heat and strain the tea into a teapot or mugs.

5. Add honey and lemon slices, if desired, for added sweetness and flavor.

6. Stir well and enjoy the warm and comforting ginger-turmeric tea.

Green Smoothie with Leafy Greens and Berries

Leafy greens, such as spinach and kale, are rich in vitamins, minerals, and antioxidants, which can be beneficial for managing gout. This green smoothie combines leafy greens with berries, which are also known for their antioxidant properties, to create a delicious and nutrient-rich beverage that can support your gout management efforts.

Ingredients:

- 1 cup packed fresh spinach or kale
- 1 cup frozen mixed berries (such as blueberries, strawberries, and raspberries)
- 1 ripe banana
- 1 cup almond milk
- 1 tablespoon chia seeds

- 1 tablespoon honey (optional)

Directions:

1. In a blender, combine the fresh spinach or kale, frozen mixed berries, ripe banana, almond milk, chia seeds, and honey (if using).
2. Blend on high until smooth and creamy.
3. Taste and adjust sweetness with more honey, if desired.
4. Pour into glasses and serve immediately for a nutrient-rich and refreshing green smoothie.

Hibiscus Tea with Lime and Mint

Hibiscus tea is known for its potential anti-inflammatory properties and can be a refreshing beverage to include in your gout management plan. This hibiscus tea with lime and mint is tangy and flavorful, perfect for sipping on a hot day.

Ingredients:

- 1/4 cup dried hibiscus flowers

- 4 cups of water
- Juice of 1 lime
- Fresh mint leaves
- Honey or stevia (optional)

Directions:

1. In a saucepan, bring the water to a boil.
2. Add the dried hibiscus flowers to the boiling water and remove from heat.
3. Let the mixture steep for about 10 minutes.
4. Strain the tea into a pitcher and let it cool to room temperature.
5. Once cooled, stir in the lime juice and add fresh mint leaves.
6. Sweeten with honey or stevia, if desired.
7. Chill the tea in the refrigerator for at least 1 hour before serving.
8. Pour into glasses, garnish with mint leaves, and enjoy the tangy and refreshing hibiscus tea with lime and mint.

Pineapple and Turmeric Smoothie

Pineapple contains an enzyme called bromelain, which has potential anti-inflammatory properties and can help manage gout. Combined with turmeric, this pineapple and turmeric smoothie is a delicious and healthy beverage that can support your gout management efforts.

Ingredients:

- 1 cup frozen pineapple chunks
- 1 ripe banana
- 1/2 teaspoon ground turmeric
- 1/2 teaspoon ground ginger
- 1 cup coconut milk
- 1 tablespoon honey (optional)

Directions:

1. In a blender, combine the frozen pineapple chunks, ripe banana, ground turmeric, ground ginger, coconut milk, and honey (if using).
2. Blend on high until smooth and creamy.

3. Taste and adjust sweetness with more honey, if desired.

4. Pour into glasses and serve immediately for a tropical and nutrient-rich pineapple and turmeric smoothie.

Chapter 9: Meal Planning and Tips for Gout-Friendly Eating

In this chapter, we will delve into the importance of meal planning and provide practical tips for creating gout-friendly meal plans. We will explore the key components of a gout-friendly diet, including the types of foods to include and avoid, portion sizes, meal timing, and hydration. We will also discuss strategies for grocery shopping, meal prepping, dining out, and managing special occasions while adhering to a gout-friendly diet. By the end of this chapter, you will be equipped with valuable insights and practical strategies to incorporate into your daily routine for effective meal planning and gout-friendly eating.

Understanding the Components of a Gout-Friendly Diet

A gout-friendly diet typically emphasizes consuming foods that are low in purines, a compound found in many foods that can contribute to the production of uric acid in the body. When purines are broken down, they form uric acid, which can accumulate in the joints and trigger gout attacks. Therefore, reducing purine-rich foods in the diet is a critical aspect of managing gout.

In addition to reducing purine-rich foods, a gout-friendly diet should also focus on other key components, such as:

1. Low-Fat and Low-Sugar Foods: Consuming foods that are low in saturated fats and added sugars can help manage weight and reduce the risk of developing other health conditions, such as obesity, high blood pressure, and diabetes, which are common risk factors for gout.

2. High-Fiber Foods: Foods that are high in fiber, such as whole grains, legumes, fruits, and vegetables, can help promote satiety, regulate blood sugar levels, and support digestive health. They are also typically low in purines, making them excellent choices for a gout-friendly diet.

3. Nutrient-Dense Foods: Opting for nutrient-dense foods, such as lean proteins, dairy or dairy alternatives, and a variety of colorful fruits and

vegetables, can provide essential vitamins, minerals, and antioxidants without contributing to excessive purine intake.

4. Hydrating Foods and Beverages: Staying well-hydrated is essential for managing gout, as it helps flush out excess uric acid from the body. Choosing hydrating foods, such as water-rich fruits and vegetables, and drinking plenty of water throughout the day can help maintain optimal hydration levels.

5. Moderation of Alcohol and Caffeine: Alcohol and caffeine can potentially trigger gout attacks, as they can increase the production of uric acid in the body or interfere with its elimination. Therefore, it is important to consume these beverages in moderation or avoid them altogether, depending on individual tolerance and triggers.

Creating a Gout-Friendly Meal Plan

Meal planning involves intentional and thoughtful selection of foods and beverages that align with the principles of a gout-friendly diet. It can help individuals with gout make informed choices and maintain a healthy and balanced diet.

Here are some practical tips for creating a gout-friendly meal plan:

1. Consult with a Healthcare Provider or Registered Dietitian: Before embarking on any dietary changes, it is crucial to consult with a healthcare provider or a registered dietitian who can provide personalized guidance based on your medical history, lifestyle, and specific needs.

2. Educate Yourself about Gout-Friendly Foods: Familiarize yourself with the types of foods that are low in purines and suitable for a gout-friendly diet. This includes foods like whole grains, legumes, fruits, vegetables, lean proteins (such as chicken, fish, and tofu), low-fat dairy or dairy alternatives, and hydrating beverages like water or herbal tea.

3. Plan Balanced Meals: Aim to create balanced meals that incorporate a variety of nutrient-dense foods from different food groups. Include a source of lean protein, such as grilled chicken or fish, along with whole grains, plenty of colorful fruits and vegetables, and healthy fats like nuts or seeds.

4. Portion Control: Pay attention to portion sizes, as overeating can contribute to weight gain, which can increase the risk of gout. Use smaller plates and bowls to help control portion sizes, and avoid eating large amounts of high-purine foods in one sitting.

5. Limit High-Purine Foods: While some purine-rich foods are essential for a healthy diet, it is important to consume them in moderation if you have gout. Foods high in purines include red meat, organ meats, seafood (such as anchovies, sardines, and mussels), and certain types of beans (such as lentils and kidney beans). Limit your intake of these foods and opt for lower-purine alternatives whenever possible.

6. Hydration: Staying well-hydrated is crucial for managing gout, as it helps flush out excess uric acid from the body. Aim to drink plenty of water throughout the day, and include hydrating foods like watermelon, cucumber, and celery in your meals.

7. Meal Timing: Pay attention to the timing of your meals, as it can impact uric acid levels. Avoid skipping meals or going for long periods without eating, as this can lead to overeating and poor food

choices later on. Aim to eat regular, balanced meals and avoid late-night snacking.

8. Meal Prep: Planning and preparing meals in advance can help you make healthier choices and avoid last-minute temptations. Set aside time each week for meal prep, such as washing and chopping fruits and vegetables, cooking grains and proteins, and packing them in portion-sized containers for easy grab-and-go options during the week.

9. Grocery Shopping: Make a list before heading to the grocery store and stick to it to avoid impulse purchases. Focus on the perimeter of the store where fresh produce, lean proteins, and dairy or dairy alternatives are typically located, and avoid the processed or sugary foods in the middle aisles.

10. Dining Out: Eating out can be challenging when following a gout-friendly diet, but with some careful choices, it is possible to enjoy a meal outside of your home. Look for options that include lean proteins, plenty of vegetables, and whole grains. Avoid fried or heavily processed foods, and ask for dressings or sauces on the side to control your intake.

11. Managing Special Occasions: Special occasions like parties or family gatherings may involve foods that are not gout-friendly. Plan ahead and make healthier choices whenever possible, but also allow yourself to enjoy small portions of treats in moderation. Focus on socializing and enjoying the company of others rather than solely focusing on the food.

12. Monitoring Progress: Keep track of your progress and make adjustments to your meal plan as needed. Monitor your symptoms, weight, and uric acid levels regularly, and work with your healthcare provider or registered dietitian to make any necessary changes to your meal plan.

CONCLUSION

As we come to the end of this journey through the world of "Delicious Recipes to Beat Gout," we hope that you have found the information and recipes shared in this book to be informative, inspiring, and most importantly, helpful in managing your gout through a healthy diet.

Gout is a painful condition that can significantly impact your quality of life. It is caused by the buildup of uric acid in the body, leading to the formation of sharp crystals in the joints, resulting in severe pain, inflammation, and swelling. While there are various treatment options available, including medications, lifestyle changes, and dietary modifications, adopting a gout-friendly diet can be a powerful tool in managing this condition.

Throughout this book, we have explored the important role of diet in managing gout and have provided you with a wide array of delicious and nutritious recipes that are designed to be gout-friendly. These recipes are packed with wholesome ingredients that are known to have anti-inflammatory properties, promote healthy digestion, and help reduce the levels of uric acid in the body, all of which can contribute to the management of gout symptoms.

From hearty breakfast bowls to flavorful lunch and dinner recipes, nutrient-rich side dishes, scrumptious snacks, and delectable desserts, we have covered a wide range of recipes that are not only designed to be beneficial for gout sufferers but are also mouthwatering and enjoyable for anyone looking to maintain a healthy lifestyle. We have also included refreshing beverage options that can complement your gout-friendly diet.

In addition to the delicious recipes, we have also provided practical tips on meal planning, portion control, grocery shopping, meal prepping, and dining out to help you incorporate these recipes into your daily routine and make sustainable changes to your eating habits. We understand that managing gout through diet requires effort and commitment, and we hope that the guidance and recipes provided in this book will empower you to take control of your health and make positive changes in your life.

It's important to remember that managing gout is a multifaceted approach that may require a combination of dietary modifications, lifestyle changes, and medical treatments. It's always best to consult with your healthcare provider or a registered dietitian before making any significant changes to your diet or lifestyle, especially if you have any underlying health conditions or are taking medications.

www.ingramcontent.com/pod-product-compliance
Lightning Source LLC
Chambersburg PA
CBHW070734250726
48662CB00004B/1535